MW01223562

tips from a British Nanny

Nanny

by Penelope Fairchild

Conari Press

Published in 2008
by Conari Press
with offices at
500 Third Street, Suite 230
San Francisco, CA 94170
www.redwheelweiser.com

Copyright © Complete Editions 2008

All rights reserved. No part of this work may be reproduced or utilised in any
form or by any means, electronic or mechanical, including photocopying,
recording or by any information storage and retrieval system, without the prior
permission of the publisher.

First published in the United Kingdom in 2006
exclusively for Marks & Spencer plc

ISBN 978-1-57324-416-9

Cover and design by Peter Wilkinson
Illustrations courtesy of the Beryl Peters Archive
Typeset by David Onyett, Publishing & Production Services, Cheltenham
Printed in China

Introduction

So many aspects of children's behaviour never really change over the years, but for each new generation of parents who are experiencing them for the first time they are baffling and worrying. Each chapter of this book addresses specific areas of parental anxiety, which tend to crop up with predictable regularity at particular stages of a child's development. Nannies are generally able to be fairly objective about our charges and we tend to have insights that parents do not share while they are in the thick of it. This kind of time-honoured wisdom will be invaluable to a parent who does not have the benefit of a Mary Poppins in the house.

Baby Days

For new parents the arrival of their first baby is exciting and terrifying in equal measure. So much to plan, so much equipment to buy, so much conflicting advice. With my long experience of babies, I really feel that I have seen it all before, many times, and I know that problems pass and almost all children reach their milestones at roughly the same time. I can tell you what invariably seems to work, and I hope that my advice will take some of the worry out of the early days of parenthood.

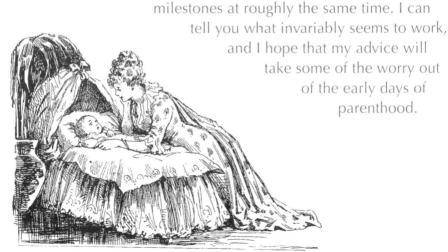

Equipment

There is so much equipment to choose from. What are the essentials?

Keep it simple, and, where possible, aim for items that serve more than one purpose (for example, travel cots that double up as playpens). It is a good idea to decide on your major items – cot, stroller, car seat – as early as you can, so that you can order them in good time. This will also give you the chance to get the cot set up, and practise installing the car seat and putting the stroller up and down so that you feel a bit more confident when the baby arrives. It may

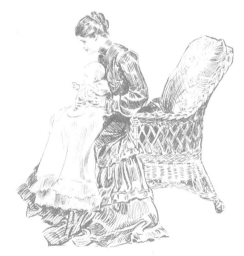

be a good idea to choose the kind of cot that converts into a little bed later, but in any case, choose the sturdiest model you can find, with adjustable base levels. A Moses basket and stand is not essential, but may be very convenient if your baby is going to spend time sleeping in your bedroom.

The nursery and sleeping

I want my baby to sleep in our room at first. Will this cause problems later?

Even if you have your baby in your room at night – which is quite likely, at least at first – you should get them used to the nursery from the start. Settle babies in the nursery at nap time, and after their bath, so that they get used to the room and like being there. That way you will not be transferring them to an unfamiliar place at three or six months, and they will probably find it easier to settle in the room more permanently.

Nanny's tips for furnishing the nursery

- Have a comfy chair in the room – not a rocking chair for safety reasons. Any self-respecting toddler will try to pull themselves upright on the furniture, so it all needs to be sturdy and secure.
- Make it as dark as possible so that you can at least try to

discourage early waking. You need black-out blinds or
curtains with black-out lining, and if you have curtain poles,
have a pelmet that goes right down over them. If you can
avoid even a chink of light you may avoid your baby joining
in with the dawn chorus.

- Put in a dimmer switch or night light so that you can settle
them down in a cosy light.
- Fitted carpets are safer than rugs if you are dashing into the
dark room in the middle of the night.

Feeding and weaning

Should I demand feed my new baby, or stick to a routine?

If you are breast-feeding your new baby some people favour
demand feeding whenever the baby cries for food. This can make
your life much easier in some ways, but it does mean that your life
is ruled by your little baby, and it can be very difficult to fit
demand feeding a second or third baby around the needs of older
children.

I recommend a compromise where you introduce the elements of a
four-hourly routine into breast-feeding, but remain adaptable to

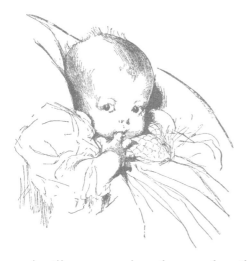

your baby's needs as well. After all, the idea of four-hourly feeding comes from expert observation of a baby's needs. In my experience, even a demand-fed baby will have arrived at approximately four-hourly feeds by about six weeks old.

Babies do like sucking, and will go on and on for comfort if you let them. This applies equally to bottle- and breast-fed babies, but for breast-fed babies just the smell of breast milk is enough to make them cry, so mothers offer them a little feed to soothe them. Of course, this is fine, but if you do it all the time you will be exhausted.

Is there any limit on how long a baby should feed for?

My feeling is that breast-feeding mothers should try to be firm, and allow ten minutes each side which should be enough as long as baby does not become genuinely hungry between feeds, when you might need to go on for a little longer at feed times.

As a rule, for both breast and bottle, I think you should put aside about half an hour for a feed, to include a diaper change and settling afterwards.

What do you feel about breast-feeding in public?

Your baby's needs must come first, and if you are out and about together and the baby has not been fed for four hours and is hungry, then that is your priority. I think mostly mothers manage to be fairly discreet about this. Other people are certainly much more tolerant these days, and quite right too. I would say, though, that feeding in a public place is not as peaceful as sitting at home, and I can imagine which the baby prefers. Wherever you are, though, I think you just have to make yourselves as calm and comfortable as possible.

Do I need to make changes in my life to breast-feed successfully?

These days nobody seems to look after new mothers the way I think they should. When I was starting out as a maternity nanny we would always make sure that our Mums had three square meals every day, with a lot of water to drink and plenty of rest, and I still think that is a good policy. I must say that calm and rested mothers are likely to be the ones with contented babies, so accept any help you are offered, and make things as easy for yourself as you can, especially in the early days of breast-feeding.

If your baby is not settling well to breast-feeding I recommend spending half an hour before the feed relaxing with the baby, to help you both get into a calm mood.

I am worried that I won't be able to breast-feed. Will bottle-feeding harm my baby?

I have looked after breast- and bottle-fed babies, and in my experience they all do just fine. If, for some reason, you can't breast-feed then don't worry, a bottle-fed baby will get good nutrition from formula milk, and will still be just as cosy and comfortable in your arms.

Nanny's tips for feeding

- Don't have visitors in the room during a feed – it can be very distracting for a baby.

- Bottle-feeding can be as cosy for a baby as breast-feeding if you hold the baby close and comfortable.
- You don't have to jiggle the baby around after a feed. Wind will come up of its own accord.

Weaning

When should I start to wean my baby?

Weaning – breast to bottle to food, or bottle to food – is a gradual process that usually starts at around six months or so. The important thing is to take your time. Don't panic if your baby doesn't get interested in food as soon as others the same age; they generally all start to level out by the time

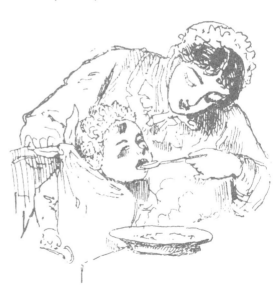

they are about one year old. Milk is the main nutrient until they are 12–14 months old.

Nanny's tips for weaning

- Slowly introduce tiny tastes of simple, fresh, organic food, starting at a time of day when your baby is in a good mood, not tired or over-hungry.
- Get them to try using a feeding cup from quite early. This encourages independence, but it can be messy to start with. Give them a cup of water to drink while they are in the bath: they can make lots of mess here and it won't matter.
- Start your baby on the kind of food you want them to eat when they are a bit older.

Routines

You need to impose a structure on your day with a baby; you will feel in control and the result of that is that your baby will feel more secure. Comfort and security for children comes in part from knowing when it is time to eat, play, bath or sleep. A good routine will establish patterns of eating and sleeping that will stand you all in good stead. It is best if a routine develops fairly organically. Start with a regular nap or meal time and fit in with your own routine and lifestyle. Children like consistency.

How can I establish a routine?

By the time your baby is three or four months old you will notice some patterns emerging. Babies will be sleepy at some times, alert and lively at others, and will generally have some regular feeding times. By six months they will usually wake up at about the same time each day and eat at predictable times. You need to capitalise on this, and, starting from a fixed point in the day, gradually work out a routine. If your baby is waking at roughly the same time each day then you can start an official breakfast time, and all will follow on from there. Have some time to play, followed by a morning nap, a little outing and an early lunch. If you can, then get them straight into an afternoon nap, which can last for up to two hours. If this gets too late, it will affect bedtime, so try to have it straight after lunch. After the nap, another little outing, perhaps to a friend's house, followed by supper, bath and bedtime. And there you have a perfect day for a baby.

How should I settle my baby for a nap? He usually dozes off in his stroller when we are out, but will hardly ever sleep in his cot in the daytime.

Your baby will often let you know he is tired – signs include being a bit grumpy, putting his head on one side or rubbing his eyes. If you see any of these signs, put him in his cot rather than rushing out with the stroller. If he makes a fuss about being in the cot go in and comfort him without picking him up, then try again to leave him there. If you can persevere, this should work after a while.

If you need to wake him up from his nap to go out, then try stroking his back gently and chatting to him before picking him up for a lovely cuddle. When you get the routine established he may well start waking automatically at about the same time each day.

A six-month-old baby is starting to stay awake for longer in the day, so there is lots of time to play and enjoy his company, but if you are to get anything done, you will welcome the establishment of regular nap times.

Nanny's tips to help you establish your nap-time routine

- A musical toy can help baby recognise that it is nap time.
- When you have established a nap time try to stick with it and don't book doctor's appointments or social things at those times – stick to times when you know your baby is usually alert for these.
- Keeping a diary will help you to track your progress.

Bedtime routine

It is really important to establish a bedtime routine for your baby. By the time they are around six months old most babies are quite capable of sleeping through the night, but the fact is that a lot of them don't. Sad to say, this is at least partly because parents love their little babies so much that they don't let them learn to get to sleep on their own. When you are in the exhausting early stages of parenthood it is so tempting to do whatever is easiest to settle your baby to sleep – rocking, cuddling or letting them fall asleep while feeding – but if they can learn to put themselves to sleep at a young age you will all be much happier.

Nanny's tips for a good night's sleep

- Make sure the room is the right temperature – around 16–21C/ 62–70F.
- Invest in a good baby monitor and always remember to turn it on.
- Steer clear of cot bumpers, pillows (until at least age one) cuddly toys and superfluous bedding because of the dangers of overheating and suffocation.
- Babies often wake up in the night because they have kicked off their blankets and are cold. From about three months old you could try a baby sleeping bag, an all-in-one fitted garment that fits on over their nightclothes

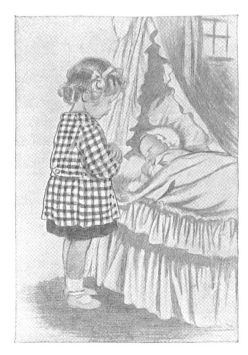

and leaves room to kick at the bottom while removing the need for covers.

- When babies are at the stage of standing in the cot, change to a sleep suit with legs at the bottom so they don't trip up.
- If you prefer blankets, put the baby towards the bottom of the cot so that they won't slip down right under the blankets in the night.
- This is easier for a nanny than for a mother, I know, but to settle baby down I recommend daily use of a musical mobile above the cot at bedtime. Turn it on, tuck them in, say goodnight and go. If they get to know this routine likely as not they will oblige by going to sleep.

Bathing and changing

I like to give a baby a bath every day and they generally seem to enjoy it. It must feel quite a natural environment for a new baby; if they do make a fuss at bath time it could be that they are not being held right or don't feel safe.

What is the safest way to bath a new baby?

You will need a baby bath. You can get a bath with a stand, or one that fits in or over your bath, which will be easy to fill using the shower attachment. I favour a foam bath support, which fits in the baby bath, and helps baby to feel supported and safe. Bath water for a newborn baby should be body temperature. To check it, it should not feel hot or cold when you dip your elbow or the side of your hand in the water, but the same temperature as your body. Get into the habit of running the cold water in first, as this is the best thing to do to avoid scalding when you graduate to the big bath.

How often should I wash my baby's hair?

You can give their hair a gentle rinse every day in the bath. It is more a matter of rinsing off any encrusted food with some warm water than a serious wash. If you do decide to use baby shampoo, be very sparing and dilute it a lot as even mild detergent can be a challenge to a little baby's delicate skin. Dry the baby's head by rubbing very gently with a cloth diaper, and make sure the ears, and behind the ears, are completely dry.

Nanny's tips to make bath time happy and safe

- Make sure you have assembled everything you need before

you start – you cannot leave baby alone in the water even for a second.

- Check that the bathroom is nice and warm.
- You will need a soft face cloth or sponge, gentle unperfumed soap or baby bath liquid, a bath towel with a hooded corner, a soft muslin to dry the baby's face, bath toys, baby hairbrush, diaper paraphernalia and clean clothes.
- Even little babies can enjoy playing in the bath; they love having water trickled onto their tummies with a sponge from very early on. When they graduate to toys, they will like things like a squeaky rubber duck, or a plastic cup or bottle. Make sure you avoid sharp edges – everything is put in their mouths.
- Hold your baby firmly in the bath.

Dressing

You need to stock up on the basics for a new baby, but don't buy too much because you will probably be given lots of clothes as presents once the baby arrives. Try not to buy things that are much too big at this stage; it is likely to be a bit uncomfortable for the baby.

Tips from Nanny

Nanny's tips for a well-dressed baby

- A baby's clothes should not be restricting or uncomfortable, or hard to put on or take off.
- Only put things over a baby's head that will go easily. If the neck opening is not large enough and you have to force the garment then don't keep it. Babies and children hate things being pulled over their heads.
- Summer and winter I would always put a little baby in a vest – the kind with poppers between the baby's legs that ensure there are no gaps. Little babies can't move around to get warm, so a vest is usually a good idea.
- Babies lose a lot of heat through their heads, so put a little bonnet on a winter baby.
- If you are using bootees or socks make sure that they are not too tight as the bones in their toes are still soft and easily damaged.
- I like to let toddlers have bare feet when they are indoors until they are confident walkers as it helps them not to slip.

How can I be sure that I have got the right amount of clothing on my baby?

It is more common for babies to be over-heated from being over-wrapped than for them to be too cold – and it is more dangerous. You can tell if a baby is too hot: they will have red faces, sweaty hands and heads and they feel exceptionally hot when you pick them up. If they are left to sweat too much they can get dehydrated and over-heating can make them lethargic and sleepy so they may not cry to let you know they are too hot. It is a matter of common sense really. Look at the weather, think about what you are wearing, and dress your baby accordingly. If you take your baby into somewhere that is significantly hotter than the temperature outside and you are taking off a layer of clothes yourself, do the same for your baby.

Baby Blues

This is a worrying, exhausting and hormone-charged time alongside the joy of the new baby, so don't be surprised by your feelings. If you think that you or someone you know has tipped over into full-scale depression contact your GP. Otherwise talk to people about how you are feeling, and try not to feel guilty or pressured.

Nanny's calming tips for baby and mum

- Soothing music such as lullabies or a bit of Bach or Mozart go down well with babies.
- Cuddle and rock baby. Try baby massage, and get a lovely relaxing massage for yourself.
- Try a drop of camomile or lavender oil in your bath.
- Pop baby in the pram and go out. A walk in the fresh air will do you both good.
- Meet other mothers and babies. This is an invaluable support network for you and will provide the babies with instant playmates as they get older.

Toddlers

Capricious, exasperating, demanding and utterly charming, toddlers are exploring the world around them with a vengeance. They take their lead from you in so much, and develop so fast that it will repay you to be ahead of the game, with plans to avoid the pitfalls before they happen.

Eating

Children in the toddler age group can be immensely conservative in their tastes – if you let them. I always encourage my charges to try tiny amounts of many different foods from a very early age. I let them know that I think something is delicious and we try it together. I think that all sitting down together to a meal is very important in this context, and so I always eat with the children. Even if it is not really my meal time I sit down with them and have a little – I can always eat less later.

How can I encourage my toddler to eat a varied diet?

You want your toddler to be eating well-balanced meals using fresh ingredients, with lots of fruit and vegetables and a good amount of meat, fish and dairy foods. It can be worrying if their likes and dislikes threaten to unbalance the good diet that you want them to have, but there are ways of sneaking in the things they refuse. Often I find that it is texture more than taste that bothers a child. If, for instance, they find eggs slimy then I will find a way of incorporating eggs – a little cheese omelette, perhaps or that perennial favourite, pancakes – that they find palatable. I always listen to their likes and dislikes and would never force a child to eat anything. That is a sure way of putting them off completely.

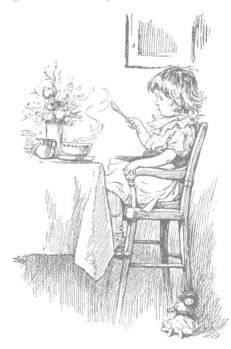

Tips from Nanny

How can I get a reluctant eater interested in food?

You can make food seem more attractive to a reluctant eater by serving it in party boxes or in unusual dishes and bowls. For a quick lunch or supper with plenty of variety fill lots of little dishes with things like cucumber sticks, cherry tomatoes, chunks of cheese and little slices of cold chicken or ham. Then let the children help themselves, making sure they take some of everything. They get a feeling of control from choosing their own food, and will probably eat more than usual. The other thing that I find often enraptures poor eaters, once they are old enough, which is usually from about two and a half to three, is to help with preparing meals. They feel so proud when they have 'cooked' something that they are much more likely to want to eat it.

Nanny's tips for happy and successful mealtimes

- Make sure that everyone has washed their hands before they sit down at table.
- It is important to be sure that everyone is sitting comfortably. Check that your child is at the right height for the table, is

not slipping down in the highchair, or, later, has not outgrown it. Children keep growing and things can change without your noticing.

- Always encourage politeness, but for little children the only important table manners are to do with safety – not having too much in your mouth because you could choke, being very careful about how you use your knife, and so on.
- Never force children to finish what is on their plates; simply clear away and go on to the next thing.
- A bit of mess really doesn't matter.

Should you give children snacks between meals?

Children often will fancy a little something between meals; it is up to you to make sure that they don't fill up on rubbishy foods that do them no good and take away their appetite for their proper meals. But, for instance, a piece of fruit and a drink of water or juice half way through the morning is fine, especially if you sit down at the table too and have your cup of coffee with them. I have often found that snack time is a good, no-pressure moment to introduce new food. If you both share cut-up fruit or a new raw vegetable at this point they may well be happy to try what you are having with no compulsion to finish it up. Incidentally, I think it is very important that they always sit down to have their snack. Children should not get into the habit of wandering around with food or drink: it could be dangerous, it will almost certainly be messy and it is quite unnecessary.

What age is the right age to stop using a highchair?

Sometime between 15 and 20 months some children will start trying to climb out of their highchair. This, and the fact that they may not even physically fit into it any more, is a sign that it is time to move into a long-legged chair or a booster seat that fixes securely to a regular seat and puts them at a comfortable height at the regular table. They will be excited at this grown up 'promotion' and will need some supervised practice at getting in and out of the chair.

My toddler is a really messy eater. Can I do anything about this?

Making a huge mess at mealtimes is a very natural part of the toddler stage. They have to learn to feed themselves and, depending on the child, this is bound to be a process of trial, error and exploration for a while. Some children learn how to do this quickly, some take ages. Your job is not to get into a state about the mess and to work out some damage limitation. For a start, keep anything to do with eating within a small, defined and easily wipe-able area. Let your child have their own little feeding spoon as soon as they take an interest, but go on doing most of the spoon-feeding yourself, or nothing much is going to end up in their mouth to start with. Make sure that children's spoons have short handles so they don't poke themselves in the eye. Put a big plastic

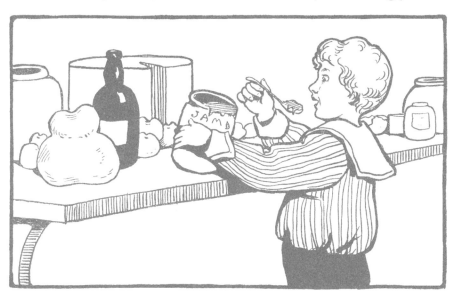

sheet under the highchair, invest in a supply of bibs and let them get on with it.

What do you think about sweets?

If you forbid sweets and chocolate you make them immensely attractive to the child, so I would never do that, but I do think you have to have some rules around this issue. It is best if you are in charge of the sweets, and you decide when they can be eaten, preferably infrequently, in very small quantities, and only after a meal, because if eaten before they really can spoil a child's appetite. Of course however successful you are at keeping to rules like this with your first child, younger siblings are going to want sweets and chocolate they see the older ones having, and it does get more difficult then.

Nanny's tips to avoid faddy eating

- Eat with your children when you can – they learn how to behave at table and enjoy the social aspect of a meal.
- Don't answer the phone during mealtimes. Take them with you if the doorbell rings. Don't leave them alone with food; there is always a danger that little children can choke.

Tips from Nanny

- They need lots of water (not fizzy drinks and only diluted fruit juice). Put water in a colourful plastic bottle and they will drink it happily.
- Young children are often daunted by a big helping of food. Give them small portions, with 'seconds' if they want.
- Stick to healthy snacks. Keep sweet and salty snacks for parties and treats.
- If they are difficult about eating don't make mealtimes a battle – you won't win.
- Get them involved when you blend juices and smoothies, and let them 'help' you with some of the food preparation; this really encourages poor eaters to take more of an interest in their food.
- Keep different components of the meal separate on their plates; they often hate it if things are mixed up.
- Don't be too obsessive about anything to do with food: children will pick up on it and become obsessive themselves. Even things like messy fingers or faces, which are quite natural and unavoidable, can worry them if you always make a fuss.

Sleeping

I have heard parents say, with more than a twinge of guilt, that the best time of day is when their little darlings are safely tucked up and fast asleep. I don't think they should feel guilty at all. A peaceful evening and a soundly-sleeping child should be the reward at the end of every well-spent day. Unfortunately, in the real world, getting children off to bed and sleeping through the night can be a real

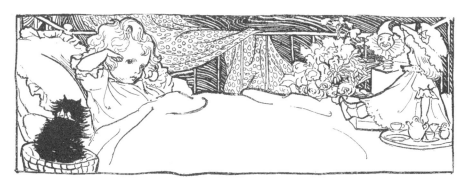

problem for many parents. Just like adults, some children are larks, some children are owls, some need less sleep than others. Two siblings can have very different sleep patterns and needs. You just have to find a way to accommodate their needs in a schedule that suits you all. It seems to me that the more sleep children have, the more they want, so it is a waste of time to keep them up late in the hope that they will wake later in the morning. Physically active toddlers really need a good night's sleep so that they won't be tired and grumpy the next day so you need to get them into good sleeping habits as early as you possibly can.

How do I get my children to accept a regular bedtime?

You need to establish a lovely, calm bedtime routine, that the children will actually enjoy. Start with a play in the bath (non-slip bath mat firmly in place), followed by pyjamas, tooth-brushing and then a quiet, calm time before bed. If parents get home from work at around this time I ask them not to inject excitement into the proceedings. What the child needs now is calm, undivided attention and a story in bed. This can be chosen by the child, though if you are sensible you will keep them to fairly gentle stories with no scary monsters to worry them, and should last for about 20 minutes before the light goes out. It is good if they have the story in their bedroom so that they associate the room with relaxation, cosiness and comfort. What could be nicer for a child than to snuggle up with someone they love for one of their favourite stories? It can be a magical time of day for you both. For this age group, between one and three years old, I think that from seven to at the latest eight o'clock is the right time for bed, but whatever time you decide upon, do try to stick to it. An overtired child will be harder to settle in bed and may well wake up in the night if their sleep pattern gets out of kilter.

When is the best time to move from a cot to a bed?

Children vary so much, but if you are fairly observant, you will notice the signs that tell you when your child is ready to move into

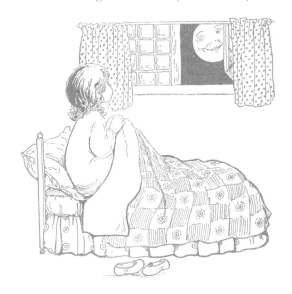

a bed. They may be 14 months or well over two; for some, you will have to make the decision for them. Often, the first sign that a move is imminent will come when they start throwing toys out of the cot. Then they will try to climb out to get them back. This can be quite a height for a baby, so you don't want them to fall. This is where the canny purchase of a cot that converts to a child bed really pays dividends. All you have to do in that case is to lower the cot mattress to a position near the ground. Lower one set of bars, and put a comfy sheepskin rug or a nest of pillows in place to soften the little fall if they roll out of bed in the night. Or just use the mattress on the floor for a while before moving on to a bed. Keep one side against the wall to reduce the possibilities for falling, and keep all the familiar bedding and soft toys from the cot for the new bed.

It is important that they don't associate the move from cot to bed with the arrival of a new baby. That on its own is quite enough change for a toddler to cope with at one time, and they might resent the baby for, as they see it, kicking them out of their cot. So, although that may well seem like a logical time to make the move, try to do it before the baby arrives or quite a long time after. The same goes for moving house. They will settle much better if as much as possible is the same as it was before the move.

Nanny's tips for a peaceful night

- Make going to bed a treat – never a punishment.
- Don't let children get over-excited in the run up to bedtime

and try to make sure they are tucked up in bed before they are too tired to get to sleep.

- Make sure that bedtime is the same every day, if you can.
- Don't let your child depend on your presence to get to sleep. This is something they need to be able to do for themselves.

What should I do about nightmares?

No matter how much you try to protect your child from frightening things they are going to have the occasional nightmare, and for some children (often, it is thought, the most intelligent ones), it is a regular occurrence. It is important that you take them seriously, and encourage the child to talk about the dream, so that you can try to reassure them.

How do you stop children wandering around the house at night?

You will sleep much better yourself if you know that your children are safe in their rooms, and you really don't want there to be any chance of them running around unsupervised in the middle of the night. I think that the best thing is to put a safety gate on the bedroom door before the child is old enough to notice it, and long before they start climbing out of bed. This is really for the child's protection.

Nanny's tips to solve night-time problems

- Listen to your child. If they are telling you about something that frightens them talk it over and respect their feelings. The worry is real to them; even if it is something like monsters in the cupboard it will keep them awake unless you can calm their fears.
- It does no harm to sit with a child, holding hands, until they drop off sometimes, or to pick them up and give them a cuddle if they have had a nightmare or are feeling ill, but if you make it a regular thing you may regret it.
- Let your child keep the bedroom door open, and have a night light in the hall if they want.
- If a child is crying in the night go straight to see what is the matter. That may be enough to reassure them.

Now that my baby is eighteen months, what should we be doing about afternoon naps?

Toddlers have such busy, active lives that they still really need to nap during the day if they are not going to collapse in an emotional and over-tired heap before bedtime. It is a pivotal part of the daily routine. Ideally, what is needed once a child is past the first birthday is one long nap a day, probably after a fairly early lunch. Two hours is about the right amount of time to sleep, otherwise you may have trouble getting them off to sleep at bedtime. If you skip the nap they will probably get really tired in the afternoon and fall asleep at a time that means bedtime has to be delayed.

Tantrums

Tantrums are the unacceptable face of toddlerhood, but, alas, they are fairly inevitable, though some children do get through this stage more gracefully than others. You can't make the tantrums go away, but you can understand what is going on, and do things to make the impact of tantrums less severe. This age is full of frustrations: toddlers know what they want, or they know they want *something*, but they cannot explain it to you. It is so easy to get things wrong. I can remember a two-year-old molten with fury and grief because I had broken her biscuit in half so that she could have something in both hands. Better to give in at that stage, and provide two unbroken biscuits, because you simply cannot reason with a toddler.

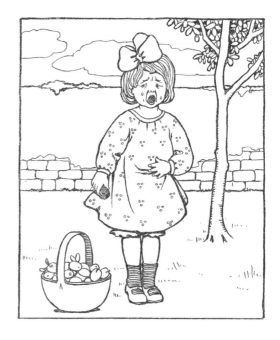

Tantrums can be made worse by change or stress, illness, over-tiredness, boredom or too much unexpended energy. Being propelled into situations they cannot cope with, or given too many choices when they are not equipped to make complex decisions can also lead to a powerful excess of emotion. So keep things simple. Ask if they would like an apple or a banana, don't give an entire fruit-bowl-worth of choices. It is good for them to feel in control of a simple decision.

My eighteen-month-old has terrible tantrums whenever I leave him at day care, which I have started to do once a week. How should I deal with this? It is very upsetting.

Separation anxiety often causes tantrums in this age group. Your son is simply afraid of being apart from you – he doesn't feel safe, because he has not yet got used to this new arrangement. That is why it is a really good idea to start very early to take your child out and about to get used to lots of other adults, children and places before they really know what is going on. They gradually build up relationships with other adults and feel safe in places other than home, and then it is much easier to leave them. It may help if you take something familiar like a toy or a favourite blanket that reminds your son of home and will help him settle. If you stay with him at the day-care center for a little while and leave when he has got involved in a game he may not notice you are gone. Otherwise, you are just going to have to weather the tantrums, taking heart from the fact that this is a very normal stage and, ghastly as it is, it will pass.

Nanny's tips for surviving tantrums

- It is impossible to reason with a toddler. Best to remove them from a problem straight away, and distract them with something else – I always keep a bubble-blowing kit handy for those moments when a quick diversion is clearly necessary to avert disaster.

- Tone of voice is all. If they realise they have incurred your disapproval, they may remember for next time. However, getting angry back at them is never going to calm the situation down.
- Sometimes you just can't stop them from having a tantrum, but the best thing you can do is ignore it. Don't respond to a tantrum – once they learn that they get no response from this kind of behaviour they may stop of their own accord.
- Comfort them afterwards – they will probably feel horrible after all that excess of emotion.
- Don't go into battle with them about everything – it is horrible to have to say no all the time. You can give in to some daft requests that will make them happy and put your foot down about the things that really can't be done.
- Always try to offer an alternative to a doomed request. "Granny won't want you to bounce on her new sofa, but she would love it if you help her to pick some strawberries in the garden."

Potty training

Don't rush into potty training before your child is ready. In all probability, the later you leave it the quicker it will be. Children only really become aware that there is a voluntary aspect to bodily functions at about 18 months, so there is really no point in starting any earlier.

How will I know when to start potty training?

Sometime after they are 18 months children start to tell you they need changing when they are wet, and they may even take off their own wet diaper. At this point you can start to introduce the potty just before bath time. Get a simple plastic potty, and praise all successful attempts to use it. After a while start using the potty straight after meal times. It can take some of the pressure off the child if you include a favourite doll or teddy in the potty training process; getting them to wear a diaper, sit on the potty, and graduate to grown-up pants along with the child. Never force a child to sit on the potty. If they are reluctant, just leave it for a few days and then try again. If you have a special storybook or song tape that is just for potty time that can make it seem more fun.

My toddler is terrified of the flushing toilet. How can I get her to use it?

Lots of young children are a bit scared by flushing. They are sometimes afraid they will fall down the toilet and be washed away, or sometimes it is just the noise that bothers them. Get them used to this by taking them in with you, letting them play with the flushing mechanism and seeing that you come to no harm. When your daughter has got over her fear, take her with you to buy her own child-size seat and little climbing stool so that she can use the toilet herself. Always stay with her for a while to reassure her. This is a good time to get her into the routine of always washing her hands after using the loo.

Nanny's tips for painless potty training

- Wait until your child seems ready to start potty training, and never compare them with others. I have often found that if you leave it until the children are two or two and a half and virtually begging to be let out of nappies you will have a quick and relatively stress-free transition.

Tips from Nanny

- Choose a stress-free time to start – probably not when there is a new baby in the house and your toddler has enough to cope with already.
- It can be easier to start in the summer, when there are fewer clothes to bother about – but don't worry if this isn't possible.
- If your child resists the potty invite an older child round who will show off their potty skills as this may encourage your child to want to copy them.
- Don't rush them into sleeping through the night with no diaper. There is no hurry for this, and it does worry a lot of children. A good time to start is when you find that their diaper is dry most mornings, and you can practise by having diaper-less nap times first.

'Play Nicely'

Parents worry a lot about getting the 'right' toys for stimulation and learning, and often go overboard for tasteful toys – distinctly retro, made of wood, lovely to look at and universally ignored by the children. There is really no need to shower a child with masses of

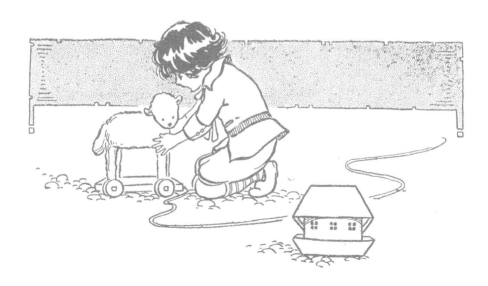

toys – particularly if they are not right for their stage of development. Give fewer toys rather than lots – if they have too many they tend to just heave them around the room rather than playing with them. Simple, everyday objects are often the very best toys – a cardboard box with a bit of string attached to pull along; a saucepan and a wooden spoon for a drum kit; or a clothes-line strung up between two chairs, so a child can peg up the contents of your scarf drawer – all these will provide hours of uncomplicated fun.

Am I choosing the right toys?

Children learn a lot from their toys, so finding the right toy, with the right play value for your child's age and stage, is important. At four months a child will be happy with a simple rattle – a few months later something a little more complex, with bits that move, will be just right. There is no point giving the more complicated toy earlier in the hope of geeing the baby along – it will just slip through her fingers and be of no interest. A ten-month-old may love to bang a drum – a younger baby might not have nearly so much fun with it. Giving a toy too early is frustrating and may mean that the child is bored with it by the time he is really ready for it.

Is that toy too young for my child?

Children develop at their own pace and you should not make them give up particular toys before they are ready. Never tell a child a toy is too babyish for them – that is bad for their confidence. You will know when they have grown out of a toy; they just won't play with it any more. Children tend to work out each stage of development for themselves, and you should try and leave them to it rather than forcing the pace. They start to learn about sharing and co-operating when they want to play with something that needs two people. A child forced to share is often less good at it than one who decides for himself.

You should always take notice of the age recommendations on toy packaging for safety reasons, but not so much for play value. Manufacturers often seem to put ages that are really too young on their toys.

How can I organise the toybox so that we are not drowning in a sea of toys?

Always put away the toys that don't interest the child any more – which are the ones that are just lying around. Bring them out again if a younger child comes to tea and your child will be happy to see

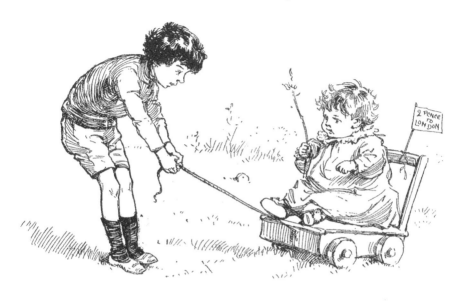

them again. Put all the day's toys away at night (helped by children who are old enough) and get out two or three different ones for any younger children for next morning's play. Don't try to restrict the use of the favourite toys they play with all the time. It should be their choice. Don't have too many toys. Parents love their children so much that they just can't resist buying them things – but children get much more fun out of having a few things that they really enjoy.

What should I do about toy safety?

The main danger in the nursery is that children may be harmed by swallowing things; so watch them all the time. People should use some common sense. It is ridiculous to give a child a toy with sharp edges or one that is easy to pull apart, with small pieces that could be swallowed. Most children begin walking aged between one and two and often fall over a bit at this stage. Be careful not to let them walk around with pencils, sharp sticks or toys like recorders until they are sure on their feet. Really children should not have pencils, except under supervision, until they are five. So many injuries can happen to children play fighting with pencils or walking with them in their hands and then tripping up. It is harder to stick to all this when younger siblings come along, but remember that small children tend to put things in their mouths and keep a strict watch.

Nanny's tips for happy playtime

- Put toys away so that the children don't have the chance to get bored with them, and bring out a few different ones every day.
- Home-made toys that let a child use some imagination can

give them a lot of fun. Always hang on to usefully sized cardboard boxes – you never know what they may turn into.

- Always have some paints and craft materials to hand – and don't worry about a bit of mess.
- Make sure a child doesn't have any toys that are aimed at an older age group. This can be very frustrating for them.
- Let children work out how to play with things for themselves, unless they ask you to help them.

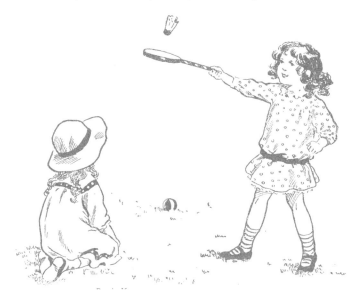

Sharing and joining in

My three-year-old is normally sociable, but finds it very hard to share toys at nursery. What can I do?

If sharing is still causing problems at this stage, it may be that your child simply hasn't had enough practice. Start in the playground, where they will have to wait their turn for the swings and slides, and will want to fit in with the other children and be accepted. Invite other children to the house to play, and if your child is finding it hard to share their precious toys suggest that you all play a game together, for which you will need to use their toys, and then thank them and praise them for letting you use them.

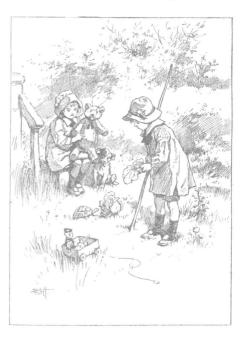

Nanny's tips for encouraging sharing

- By the time they are three or three and a half, toddlers should be able to share toys and take turns without too much fuss. You will probably need to supervise the play, especially with new children, and make sure all is going along smoothly.
- If there are problems sharing a particularly prized toy, suggest each child has five minutes to play with the toy.
- You can practise sharing by using an egg timer so that each child can have a certain amount of time on each toy. They may well find they prefer operating the timer to playing with the toy.

Good Behaviour

Good manners are really all about showing consideration for other people, but this is not something that you can expect to come

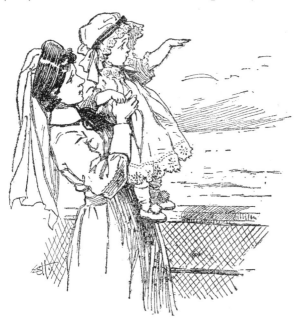

naturally to little children. They learn almost everything by example – the example that you, as parents, set. If you always treat them with courtesy and respect you should be able to expect the same back from them.

Tips from Nanny

Nanny's tips on how to teach consideration and good manners by example

- Be consistent in your rules, and make sure that everyone who looks after your children knows what the rules are.
- Always think about the example you set. Let your children see you treating others with consideration. If you offer your seat to an elderly person on the bus, explain why you are doing it, and encourage them to do the same when they are big enough.
- Praise them whenever they do something kind and thoughtful for someone else.

At what age should children start saying 'please' and 'thank you'?

Toddlers are quite ready for the kind of simple good manners that make everybody's life more pleasant. If you always say 'please' and 'thank you' they will almost certainly copy your example, and, if not, you should constantly remind them – though don't turn it into a nag. A good game that will help your toddler get the hang of things is to pass Teddy back and forwards between the two of you, saying "Please can you pass Teddy?" and "Thank you very much" at each turn.

Are thank-you letters important these days?

Once they are old enough, children should always be persuaded to write a little thank-you letter if someone has been kind enough to send them a present. Apart from anything else, the sender has no way of knowing whether or not the lovely present has arrived safely if the child doesn't trouble to thank them for it. When they are younger, you can write the letter for them and get them to add a personal touch like a little drawing.

How can you overcome shyness?

A lot of people are shy. It is a perfectly natural characteristic, but by the time we are adults most people learn how to deal with it so that it is not socially disabling. Little children have learned none of these skills, and some adults can

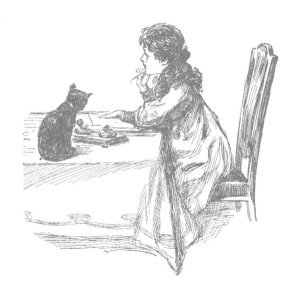

misunderstand a shy child, thinking that they are unfriendly or unsociable. Whenever I have looked after a shy child I have tried to be very understanding. I tell them that it is fine to feel shy, but that if they can make a big effort and smile at people who talk to them, it won't matter so much if they can't quite manage to talk much back. With a shy child I always support them in social situations as much as they need, and I usually find that gradually, as they get used to things, they need me less. Starting school can be hard for shy children, so encourage them as much as you can to make friends on a one-to-one basis, by having children home for tea.

Do you think table manners still matter?

As with all 'manners', behaving well at table is really about consideration for other people, and this is always going to be important. As children emerge from the relative anarchy of learning to feed themselves you can steer them by small stages into the kind of behaviour you find acceptable.

Nanny's tips for teaching good table manners

- Don't overload children with do's and don'ts, keep it simple and stick to what is important at every age.

- By the time they are about three children should be able to help set and clear the table, under your supervision.
- Hands should always be washed before a meal.
- The table is a place for pleasant conversation; no shouting, fighting or food throwing. No exceptions to these few rules and no pudding for persistent offenders. Once they realise what is at stake they will usually behave.
- Always remember 'please' and 'thank you'.
- Children should ask if they may leave the table at the end of a meal, not just wander off when they have finished eating.

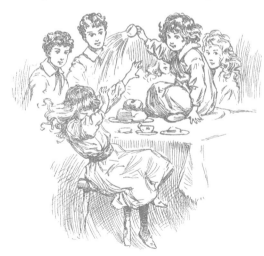

I am afraid my daughter is being bullied at her primary school. What should I do?

First, you must get her to talk to you. Children often feel that they must keep quiet about this sort of thing and suffer in silence when someone is persistently nasty to them, but that is so wrong. Keep very calm, but let her know that you are on her side and want to help to sort things out. Talk to the teacher, and see if they are aware of the situation. They may have a policy for dealing with bullying, but if nothing happens you should talk to the other child's parents. Don't be angry, but let them know that you expect them to deal with the situation. After all, you would want to intervene if your child was the culprit.

Nanny's tips for dealing with aggressive and bullying behaviour

- People encounter bullying, mental and physical, throughout their lives: I really think it helps if you learn how to overcome it in childhood.
- I am not a great believer in the 'stiff upper lip' for little children. I would always encourage my charges to tell me if

they were miserable because they felt they were being bullied; when they are small they should not have to cope alone.

- If it persisted, and the teacher was not doing anything effective about it, I would have a word with the bullying child's mother or nanny, or even with the child. Aggressive behaviour should be nipped in the bud, and any right-thinking parent or carer will want to do this.
- Someone who is being a bully at school is quite likely to be meeting with aggression or disruption elsewhere themselves – often at home. It is worth pointing this out to your child, so that they don't take it quite so personally.
- One thing that I have often found effective is to invite the bullying child to tea to see if the two could become friends out of the context of school or kindergarten. Of course, this will only work if your child thinks they can cope with it.

How do you deal with bad behaviour in the toddler age-group?

You have to make it clear, even to a toddler, that rudeness will not be accepted. Whether it is directed towards you, or other people, you should deal with it straight away, otherwise it can make your child unpopular with other adults, or children their own age, who can be surprisingly judgemental. Try to make any punishment that you feel is needed short-lived, help your child to say 'sorry', which does not always come easily, and then move on as quickly as possible. With a phase of toddler bad behaviour that you cannot see a cause for, a gold star chart for good behaviour may be much more effective than constant punishment and negativity. It is worth thinking about whether the child is being set a bad example, for instance by older children or by watching television programmes that are too grown up for them. It is always best to watch television with your child, so you know exactly what they are exposed too. However tempting it is to

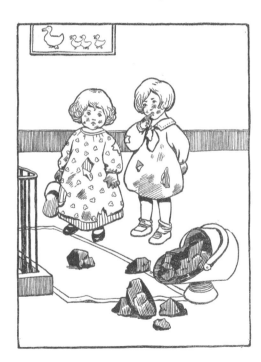

use the television as a child-minder, it is a very bad idea with this age group, particularly if they have access to the remote control.

How can I stop my children from fighting each other?

It is normal for children to squabble, but they have to do it without resorting to any kind of physical violence. You need to make very clear rules about this, and enforce them. Violence, however slight, is not the way to solve problems, and they need to be clear on that. Your rules need to encompass the little sneaky bits of sibling violence that tend to escalate into full-blown fighting, so no pinching, hair pulling or sly hitting. No exceptions and removal of a privilege or treat for any rule-breaking. Encourage better behaviour with rewards for not fighting, try to be even-handed, and always remember that the child who makes the most noise about an alleged incident may well be the one who started it.

Nanny's tips for good discipline

- Deal with rudeness or bad behaviour straight away – a toddler won't understand if you defer a rebuke.
- Bad behaviour that is allowed to continue may become a habit.

- Get down to your child's level, look them straight in the eyes and explain that they must not speak this way to people/pull their friend's hair, or whatever the offence has been, and that they have made you upset by what they have done.
- If they have been very naughty, take away the toy they are playing with, or stop what they are doing and tell them to sit still and think about what they have done (not for too long) and then help them to say 'sorry'.
- If they have been rude to another adult, or upset another child, get them to draw a picture for them, or do something else that will please them, and then make it clear that the bad behaviour incident is over. Try to praise them and make them feel good that they have 'sorted it all out'.

Sibling rivalries

A new baby arrives in a toddler's life like a hurricane, blowing a lot of cherished certainties off track. You need to work hard to minimise the effects of this. After all, your first-born has spent a happy time as the centre of your universe, a position from which it is hard to feel toppled. You can hardly blame them for needing a lot of attention and reassurance from you, just when you are having to stretch all your resources to deal with the new baby as well.

How do I introduce my two-year-old to her new brother or sister?

Your daughter should visit you in hospital as soon as possible after the new baby arrives, at which point the baby should be in the cot, or handed to someone else so that you can give your daughter a

lot of attention and love straight away. It is a good idea if the toddler and the new baby exchange gifts. The new baby has the advantage that you already know your toddler's tastes and can make sure the present is something they will love, and will remember as being from the baby.

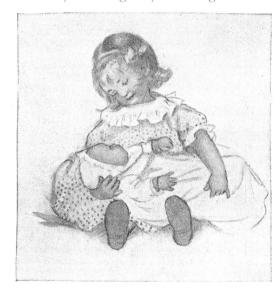

Nanny's tips for coping when the younger baby arrives

- When you bring the baby home let your partner or someone else carry them in so that you can concentrate on your toddler.
- Try not to make too much fuss of the baby in front of the toddler, and encourage the toddler to help you look after this helpless new addition to the family. Stress how useful it is to have a big child who can do so much.
- Don't leave the new baby alone with your older child. Toddlers are surprisingly strong, and the most angelic-looking little two-year-old may have murder in his or her heart at such a traumatic time.
- As soon as they develop any awareness the baby will start to worship the older child – and that generally helps.
- I think it is best to ignore a certain amount of bickering between siblings. It is irritating, but entirely natural, and you should only intervene if things get rough and there is a danger that one of them will get hurt.

Being Ill

Teething, being a bit under the weather, or being ill enough to have to go into hospital are all dreadful times for a child, and times when they really need to be able to depend on their parents. But,

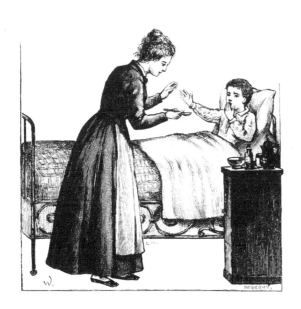

particularly in the case of illness, they are very worrying times for the parents, too. I have found that it can really help to have advice from someone who is not so directly involved.

Nanny's tips for coping with childhood illnesses

- Make a poorly child a 'nest' on the sofa so that they can be cosy and comfortable, but not feel shut away in their bedroom.
- Collect up a little basket of toys, games and things to do that you keep just for when they are ill. New song tapes can be very cheering for under-the-weather toddlers.

How will I know if my baby is ill?

You can usually just tell if your child is not well. Their behaviour is often a bit grumpier than usual, they may cry a lot or sleep for unusually long periods during the day, waking up with slightly glazed-looking eyes and a hot tummy. You can often see just from their look that a child is running a temperature. Check using a press-on thermometer for a baby, and perhaps an ear thermometer for over-twos. The normal temperature is 37C or 98.4F.

What should I do if my baby is running a temperature?

A raised temperature can be treated with Calpol, which can reduce it quickly, but let your GP know straight away if it is over 39C. Keep a record of the amount of medicine given, the time, and the

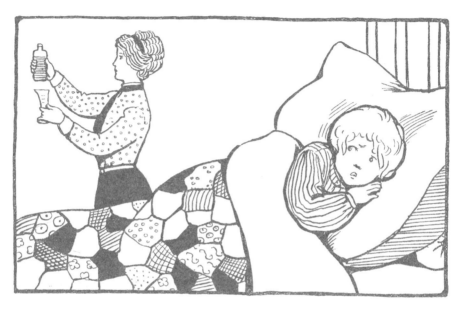

child's temperature. If the child is feverish remove clothes, sponge them down with tepid water and make sure they sip lots of cold water, as children can dehydrate very quickly when they have a fever. Don't let them curl up under a mountain of duvets however much they want to.

Tips from Nanny

Nanny's tips for helping the medicine go down

- If you can, always go for liquid medicine rather than tablets.
- If they are reluctant to take their medicine try mixing it with something very sweet, or in drinks.
- You can get a medicine syringe from the pharmacist, which may be easier to use than a spoon. If you do use one, when it is in the mouth point it at the child's cheek rather than down the throat, which could make the child choke.
- Make bribery your last resort, or you will have to think of a bribe every time they have to take any medicine.

I hear so many horror stories about teething. What can I expect to happen?

The first tooth usually arrives at some time after your baby is six months old, though it can be earlier, with the full set of baby teeth usually in place by around age two and a half. You can therefore expect some degree of teething troubles to go on from time to time for about two years, causing grouchiness, dribbles, some sleepless nights, loss of appetite when gums are sore and generally being a bit under the weather. Problems don't usually last for more than a couple of days at a time, however. If an episode that you have attributed to teething is going on for longer there may be something else underlying it, and you should consult your GP if you have any concerns.

Nanny's tips for teething troubles

- Try the old-fashioned remedy of a spot of clove oil diluted with safflower oil and rubbed on to swollen gums.
- Cold, hard food such as chilled carrot or celery stick or a piece of apple to chew and suck on may help.
- A gel teething toy which is refrigerated can be very soothing and so can a cold, damp face cloth straight from the fridge.
- Hard teething biscuits can be just the thing when they want something to bite on.
- Make sure they have plenty of fluids, especially if teething gives them an upset tummy.

Growing Up

It is very important that from an early age you encourage your children to be able to do some things for themselves. The best parenting or child care grows children who are not over-dependent on adults, whether for getting to sleep, dressing, or keeping themselves amused.

Dressing

As with so much else, the age at which children start dressing themselves entirely depends on the individual. Generally between 18 months and two years old toddlers will be able to take most of their clothes off (and will often go through a phase of doing so at inopportune moments just because they can) and by two and a half they will mostly be able to get completely dressed except for complicated buttons, zips and fastenings, for which they will still need your help.

Tips from Nanny

My son is coming up to his third birthday, but shows no inclination to dress himself. What can I do?

It may be that you have dented his confidence about dressing himself by rushing him. This often happens; we are always in such a hurry that we never think about doing things at the child's pace.

He will know he can't do things as fast as you, so he may not try for fear of making you impatient. Do things in stages, starting at the weekend, when there is no need to rush, and let him start with easy clothes that just pull on. Give him lots of praise and encouragement, and build up to letting him choose his everyday clothes, getting them ready the night before.

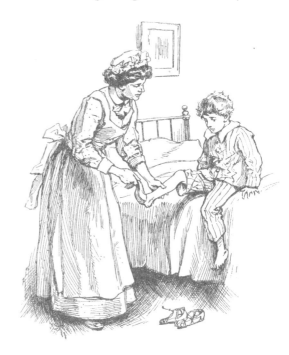

Nanny's tips for getting dressed

- Toddlers find taking clothes off much easier than putting them on, so let them start by getting themselves undressed at bath time and afterwards putting on their pyjamas, which are much easier than day clothes.

- They will start to take an interest in dressing themselves if you let them choose what they are going to wear the next day; lay it out ready for the morning. This will get you all off to a much better start than if they have to start making choices in the morning.

- Unless you are happy for your child to go to nursery dressed like a princess or superman every day, it is best to put the fancy dress and party clothes out of sight and mind at this stage or they will probably be the regular outfits of choice.

- Do praise all their efforts and choices – they will be easily disheartened if you laugh about colour or pattern combinations, however gently you do it.

- They will need your help with tricky buttons and fastenings for ages, but don't help until you are asked, and remember to say how clever they have been.

- Velcro. When it comes to shoes this saves so many child-hours each day. Leave the struggles with buckles and laces for as long as you can.

Hints of independence

Should I try to encourage my three-year-old to be a bit independent of me before she starts playgroup – and if so, how?

I like to encourage children to do things for themselves from a very early age. One of the key parts of this is letting them help around the house. There are lots of little jobs that they will enjoy doing: sorting the clean socks into pairs, setting the table, washing up (heavily supervised), tidying up toys at the end of the day. Believe me, you can turn these into fun activities, and your child will feel rewarded by praise and encouragement and will learn a lot in the process. Every time they discover a little thing that they can do for themselves, it is a big step towards independence.

Nanny's tips to encourage a little independence

- Encourage them to choose between two things, whether bedtime stories, flavours of yoghurt for pudding, colours of socks: it all helps them to be comfortable making decisions.
- Let them do things for themselves, even if it takes ages.
- Think of a new thing you want them to try – putting their

packed lunch in the lunchbox, making their own sandwich, putting dirty clothes in the laundry basket – help them with it the first time, then give them lots of praise when they do it for themselves.

- Give them a few responsibilities, such as looking after a pet.
- Allow them to make their own decisions about how to spend their pocket money – but when it's gone, it's gone.
- When they are old enough to be going anywhere without you make sure they know their address and phone number, and how to make a telephone call.
- Get them to practise asking for things in cafés and shops.

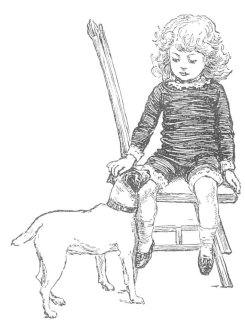

Building confidence

It is very important for a toddler to feel confident about things as they begin to go out into the world a little bit, and you can do a lot to help your child in this respect. If they are about to start nursery or playgroup, for instance, you can find out what they will be expected to be able to do, and practise a bit at home with things like hanging a coat up on a peg, eating with a knife and fork, or changing shoes. Needing help from the teacher with things like this can be a blow to a child's confidence, so a bit of practice beforehand can be very effective.

My son is two, and seems much less confident than his playmates. How can I boost his confidence?

Sometimes, and with the very best of intentions, a parent will hold a child back by helping them too much. If you are so anxious to prevent your child from failing at new things that you are always right at his side to help him, you will effectively prevent him from having any idea that he can succeed on his own. You have to step back a bit so that your son can see that you think he is capable of managing the new thing, whatever it is. Just grit your teeth and let him get on with it, and praise him for what he achieves.

Nanny's tips for boosting confidence

- Get an under-confident child to do things that you know they can succeed at, such as working out a puzzle or constructing a toy, and then praise them when they have completed it.

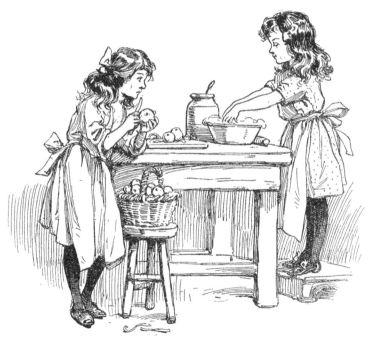

- Ask them to do a little something to help you, and give them lots of thanks when they finish the task.
- Display pictures or models they have made, and show them to other people, stressing how proud you are of them, and do all of this regularly, to help them believe in themselves.
- Don't compare a child to others their age or to siblings – the under-confident child may feel that you are getting at them even though this is far from your intention.

Starting nursery and school

Toddlers are often ready for the company and interest offered by a playgroup or nursery school by the age of two and a half to three. This is a great time to develop their social skills and get used to being in a group and away from you. It may take you both a while to get used to it, but it will make all the other separations that come later much easier. You will obviously choose your nursery or playgroup with enormous care, but the most important thing when you are looking around is to see children who are happy and well occupied.

Tips from Nanny

Can you give me some advice on how to leave my daughter at playgroup for the first time? We have never really been separated before.

This is a big moment for both of you, but you have to be very matter-of-fact about it to make it easier for your daughter. Try to get her used to being apart from you by leaving her with a friend or relation for an hour or so every few days, gradually increasing to the length of the playgroup session. Try to build up her confidence beforehand, by letting her undertake simple tasks for herself. When you first take her to playgroup see if you can go with another mother who is dropping her child for the first time, as it may be easier for two of them together. At the end of the session spend some time talking about all the things she has done, what she enjoyed the most, and what she wasn't so keen on. Give her lots of praise for doing all these new things.

Nanny's tips for starting nursery, playgroup or school with a smile

- Visit the place a couple of times with your child before they start. You may be able to spend a morning there together, but if not show them where everything is, including lockers and loos.

- Make sure they are clear about what will happen during the time they are at the playgroup, nursery or school, and discuss the amount of time they will be there in a way they understand.

- If an older sibling or friend is already there then they may be longing to move into this 'grown-up' environment, in which case things may be quite easy, but if this is not so then try to get to know a few other children who will be in the class. Invite a few over for tea and a play, on a one-to-one basis, so that some friendships can be established before your child starts.

- The teacher will be used to dealing with wobbles from new children, so once they start nursery or school you need to be very strong and say goodbye and leave them there. Don't let them see your anxiety, it can be very infectious.

- Starting this new stage can be a strain, and your child may be a bit difficult with you for a little while. It is almost a way of letting off steam for them and is usually a very short-lived phase.

Keeping them safe at home

So much to do with child safety is a matter of simple common sense, but safety-proofing your home for a first baby does require a radical new look at things. I recommend that you go round your house room by room, trying to see it from a little child's perspective. Get right down to floor level and look around. Are there any enticing sockets; dangling wires that you might try to pull yourself up on; fluttering table-cloth fringes that you could grab hold of and pull a Ming vase down on your head? Well, you get the general idea. Wires need to be securely taped back, tablecloths put away, and all the precious stuff moved well out of reach for the duration.

Nanny's tips for safety first

- Safety plugs on all electric sockets are essential. Have some spares for when you go to stay in a house or hotel that has not been child-proofed, and do be vigilant when you are out visiting. A toddler's curiosity knows no reasonable bounds.
- Install stair gates, and consider child-gates on certain doors where it may be necessary to stop them from running out of a room.

- Put safety locks on cupboards you don't want them to get into, and on windows, so that they will not open far enough for a child to get through.
- Make sure they cannot get near the oven when it is hot.
- Always check the temperature of anything you give them to eat and drink, especially if it has been microwaved.
- Cover sharp edges on furniture that is at toddler head height.
- Tape back dangling cables and knot curtain strings or lamp cords and put them out of reach.
- Have a sturdily fixed fireguard for all open fires and any gas or electric fires that they could get too close to, and turn the radiators down so that they don't burn themselves if they touch them.
- Fit door slam protectors to safeguard their fingers and fit safety film on glass doors.
- Make sure that anyone who looks after your children knows your safety rules.

Now that my little girl is walking do I need to do more safety-proofing?

A crawling baby is one thing, a perpetually inquisitive toddler quite another. As your child becomes more and more mobile, you have less and less chance of restraining her. She will soon be able to climb out of her cot, playpen and high-chair, and will probably be fascinated by stairs. As well as installing stair gates, it is important to teach her the safe way of getting down stairs, which is crawling backwards. Practise this with her – it is likely to be quite a while before she will be able to cope with stairs any other way. Try to have one room in the house that you know is completely toddler-proof, where she can play without worry, and devote some serious time to a room-by-room look at the risks in the rest of the house.

Keeping Busy
and
Having Fun

Outdoor play

It is so important to get children out in the fresh air and away from the television and the computer. The freedom they can enjoy in the park or garden and the sheer delight of running around and letting off steam are quite essential. You will never run out of things to do out of doors, and here are just a few suggestions.

Nanny's tips for things to do in the garden

- Have a scavenger hunt. You give them a list of ten or fifteen things to find in the garden – a brown leaf, a round pebble, a flower, a bouncy ball – and a little basket to put everything in, and then it is a race against time.

- Go bug-hunting with a magnifying glass and a simple book about insects which will help you all to identify your finds.
- Find a little patch of garden where your child can plant things and watch them grow. If all else fails a big plant pot or window box will do.
- Grandmother's Footsteps is a game that will keep quite a wide age range of children happy for ages.

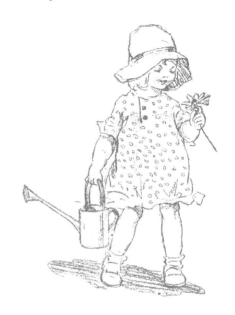

- Hopscotch, marked out with chalk on the pavement or patio, is great fun.
- Get them to help you make an obstacle course, using cushions, an empty cardboard box open at both ends, waste paper baskets to throw balls into, and anything else you can think of, and devise a course that they must complete against the clock.

Dressing up

I don't think I ever met a child who didn't enjoy dressing up. You can collect up lots of bits and pieces for a dressing up box from things you find around the house. Old hats, scarves and handbags make a start, and such essentials as cowboy hats, superman ensembles and ballet tutus can be found fairly cheaply in good

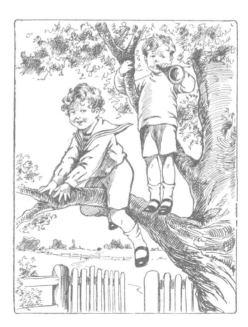

toyshops. Remember to pop the clothes through the wash every so often to freshen them up.

When they have friends to tea, give them an idea for a play to put on with you as audience, and let their imaginations run riot.

Cookery

Children always enjoy doing some cooking. There is nothing nicer on a rainy afternoon than to go into the kitchen and make some little cakes for tea. You have to supervise pretty carefully if you want edible results, but it is well worth it. Young children are always so proud that they have managed to make their own food. You should make a little book of basic fail-safe recipes for things like cakes, biscuits and cheese straws. Help them to weigh out the ingredients, and then let them mix them up in their own little bowls. Impress on them the importance of never going near a hot oven door, and that is another useful job done.

I have always found that helping to prepare meals can be a good way of encouraging a poor eater. They get so interested in the process that they actually want to eat the end results, and it can be quite a turning point.

Television

A bit of television is fine; children really enjoy 'their' programmes, and talk to each other about them. I would certainly encourage the odd half hour. But I have two rules: the set is turned off when the programme is over, and I try to watch with them, or at least to be in the room while they are watching. That way I can talk to them about the programme, and be sure I know what they are watching. I would never let the television be the 'babysitter'.

In the same way, there are some really lovely DVDs and videos for children, which I like them to sit down and enjoy as a treat on a wet afternoon rather than something that happens every day.

It is a little different for school-age children. I think that half an hour or an hour of children's television in the afternoon when they get home from school can be an excellent way for them to relax and recharge when they are tired. But, again, at the end of the programme, the television is firmly switched off. No arguments.

Nanny's rainy-day tips for playing indoors

- Start a scrapbook with photos, cuttings from magazines, birthday cards and postcards. Put in drawings, and let them dictate little stories which you can write down and add to the collection.

- Make a hidey hole with sheets draped over the furniture and camp there for the afternoon.
- Get creative with paper and paint, glitter and glue. Have an art exhibition to show off to a home-coming parent.
- Make up a dance routine to a favourite song.
- Have a tea party for favoured toys, and maybe a friend or two.

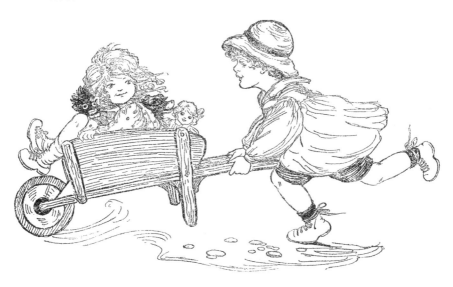

Outings and other things to do

Special expeditions to your local museum, zoo or city farm are red-letter days to be remembered, but to be perfectly honest, under-fives will derive just as much, if not more, enjoyment from much simpler outings. A picnic in the park, especially if they have helped to prepare the food and put it in a special basket, will make a toddler blissfully happy. In fact, anything that is a little deviation from routine, such as a bus ride or a visit to a café, will be full of interest for them.

Nanny's tips for happy and successful outings

- If you do go on a serious outing to somewhere busy dress the children in bright colours so that you will be able to find them in a crowd.
- Don't travel to somewhere too far away if you want to avoid over-tired grumps.
- Factor in regular stops for food and drink.
- Never, ever travel without a handy pack of wet wipes for sticky hands.

How to have Lovely Parties

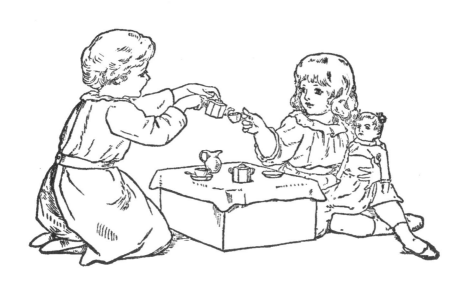

Tips from Nanny

A child's birthday party is the most important social event in the calendar, eagerly anticipated from one year's end to the next. With so much emotion riding on the occasion it can be hard to stop it ending in tears. Over the years I have organised more children's parties than I can count, so I know how to make sure that everyone enjoys themselves without going over the top.

Nanny's tips for parties for different ages

- **First Birthday** Hardly any of the young guests will be doing much at this stage so you will be catering for the grown-ups. Remember to serve cold drinks to avoid the dangers of scalding tea, and have food that won't hurt an inquisitive baby who gets hold of some. If you are serving food for the children, base it on the sort of thing your own baby actually eats, and make sure that the other mums know what there is so that little ones can't get hold of anything that they are allergic to or unused to eating.

- **Second Birthday** If you are inviting more two-year-olds than adults the safest thing is to serve their tea picnic-style, with rugs and cushions on the floor. You can make life easier by giving everyone a little food-box with a drink carton and

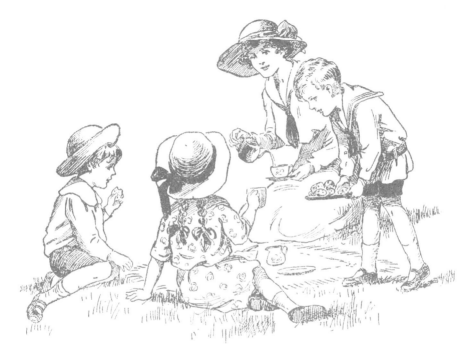

food inside. At this age they will enjoy playing with the birthday child's new toys and probably won't go for many organised games, but pass the parcel never fails. Enlist the help of a few other adults who you can depend on not to spend the time chatting while you deal with the chaos.

Tips from Nanny

- **Third Birthday** Channel all that energy with something organised like a (heavily supervised) trampolining session in the garden. It is best not to invite too many children. Between five and ten is plenty at this age. Two hours is the maximum sensible duration – make sure you put this clearly on the invitation. If anyone is going to get over-excited and behave horribly it is almost certain to be the birthday child.
- **Fourth Birthday** This is a good age to have lots of easy games. But do alternate lively ones with calm ones so that no-one gets too excited.
- **Fifth Birthday** Maybe you could go for fancy dress – possibly the last chance before they get too shy. Provide extra dressing-up clothes because some children are bound to refuse to dress up and then wish they had.

Nanny's tips for party food and drinks

- Small children probably won't appreciate masses of home cooking. Hardly anyone will eat the sandwiches, and they are all much too excited to sit down for long.
- The most successful party food for younger children is simple, small-sized and healthy. Baby tomatoes, chunks of

cucumber, little squares of cheddar cheese, a big bowl full of seedless grapes – plus cocktail sausages and crisps (you have to relax the rules a little bit for a party) is probably as much as they will eat.

- With under-fives it is probably worth avoiding chocolate as much as possible, on behavioural as well as mess-avoidance grounds.
- Home-made cupcakes and biscuits give you control over the ingredients and can look very pretty too.
- To cut down on spills juice boxes are a very good idea, and apple juice is the least staining option.

Nanny's tips for party bags

- It is worth shopping around a bit for things to put in the bags as it can be quite saddening to spend money on dreadful bits of plastic that you know will break in five minutes.
- Museum shops are a good place to hunt out inexpensive little presents.
- Make sure that you put the same things in all the bags – nothing causes more trouble than an unequal division of the spoils.

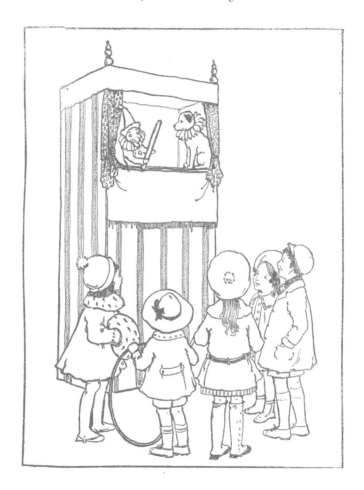

Tips from Nanny

- Don't put face paints in the bags – sometimes they can cause an allergic reaction.
- A cone of home-made popcorn is a popular home-time treat.
- A little plant in a pot that they can watch grow is something really different.